DROP

the Diet, **DROP** the

WEIGHT

DROP

the Diet, **DROP** the

WEIGHT

Secrets to
Permanent
Weight
Loss

Vera LaRee

NEW YORK

LONDON • NASHVILLE • MELBOURNE • VANCOUVER

DROP the Diet, DROP the WEIGHT

Secrets to Permanent Weight Loss

Published in New York, New York, by Morgan James Publishing in partnership with Difference Press. Morgan James is a trademark of Morgan James, LLC. www.MorganJamesPublishing.com

ISBN 9781631950049 paperback
ISBN 9781631950056 eBook
ISBN 9781631950063 audio
Library of Congress Control Number: 2020931320

Cover Concept by:
Nakita Duncan

Cover Design by:
Christopher Kirk
GFSstudio.com

Interior Design by:
Melissa Farr
melissa@backporchcreative.com

Editor: Cory Hott

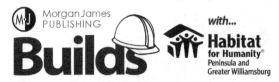

Morgan James is a proud partner of Habitat for Humanity Peninsula and Greater Williamsburg. Partners in building since 2006.

Get involved today! Visit
MorganJamesPublishing.com/giving-back

For my beautiful daughters Krisia and Meron,
who have always admired, loved, and believed in me.
I love you.

Table of Contents

Your Struggle Is Real

Lisa was desperate to lose weight and to feel better about herself. After several diets—some successful and others not so much—she seemed to gain the weight back that she lost. She loved her husband, her two children, and her job as a manager at a local IT company even though it was stressful at times. She ate more when she was stressed but didn't understand why.

Last week, she called me, nearly hopeless. Before I could finish formally introducing myself, she cried as she spoke. "I need to start a new diet … again," she said. "I stepped on the scale this morning, and the number instantly ruined my day. I knew I was gaining all the weight back that I lost last spring, but I hoped that if I quit checking the scale, the number would somehow magically stop going up. I was wrong. I hate my life right now, but I hate it more when

I'm dieting because it feels like it's on hold. I feel like I'm waiting till the diet is over or till the weight comes off to live."

She continued to cry as she went on. "The craving for food is so hard to resist at times that I cheat and screw up a lot. I feel guilty when I do though. I don't know why I do that. I should know better after all these years and diets. Sometimes after I cheat and eat bad or fattening foods, I end up eating like crap the rest of the day, but at least I promise myself to start again in the morning, right? Which I do. Usually. A lot of my diet attempts end up being epic failures though. Often when I cheat and screw up so many days in a row, I get discouraged, and I give up on the diet altogether, as I did with the last one. I went right back to eating all the bad and unhealthy food that I know is not good for me. Now look at me," she sobbed.

As our conversation continued, I learned many things about Lisa that broke my heart. She shared with me that she felt embarrassed and secretly ashamed. She loved food and couldn't seem to resist it, as she believed she should. She often wondered if she was addicted to food, especially sugar.

"Why else would it be hard for me to just quit eating it?" she said. I've read several articles about food and sugar addiction, and maybe that's what my problem is. Maybe I should give up on eating sugar." She didn't like the thought of that. She said someday she might have the willpower to give it up forever, but for now, she wanted to find a diet that would be easy to stick to.

She wondered if she should try keto again. Her friend Amanda did the keto diet and lost a ton of weight, and her other friend Mary told her that when she cut all dairy and animal products, she lost weight and felt better than ever. Lisa claimed that she tried a lot of these diets but couldn't seem to stick to them as easily as other people could.

Last spring when she lost forty pounds, she thought she was going to die. "It was torture," she said. "I don't want to go through that again, but I know I have to. I just have to." She wondered if she should try to find a new product or supplement to take but quickly decided against it. "Those darn things never do anything for me, and besides, they are usually way too expensive."

She pleaded for God to help her because she felt like such a failure. She believed she did something wrong. She asked herself, "Why does it seem like everybody else has more willpower than me?" and "Why can't I stop eating bad food and just pull myself together?" She didn't know the answers to any of her questions and continued down the rabbit hole of self-criticism. "Why can't I be lucky enough to lose weight and never gain it back?" She complained, "I still go to the gym even though I hate it, hoping that it will help keep the weight off, but I think I must not try as hard as those skinny girls. I'm lazy, and I shouldn't be. I also feel like a fat cow, and I know I am because I can see my body. Nobody needs to tell me, although I'm sure they think it when they see me."

Lisa noticed a familiar yucky feeling in the pit of her stomach when she thought that way. She told herself not to cry, that it wouldn't make her feel any better, and that it wouldn't melt the fat away.

"How can I both love food and hate it at the same time? Why can't I just eat like skinny girls, and not gain weight? They have no idea how lucky they are. When I get sad like this, food makes me feel a lot better but only while I'm eating it. Afterward, I always feel so ashamed."

Bless Lisa's heart. She tried not to care about her weight, but deep inside, she truly did care. She cared more than anybody will ever know, and the truth is that she was tired of caring so much because she couldn't seem to fix it. She went on to share how depressed she felt. She even believed her weight affected her relationship with her husband. "He says he loves me, but deep down I believe he wishes I was thinner. I don't blame him. I mean, who wouldn't want a thinner wife, right? Thinner girls just seem to have it all."

Does Lisa's story sound at all like yours? Have you, too, bought into the idea that if you could just handle suffering through a diet you will finally be free from your weight issues? Have you felt like no matter how hard you try, you can't seem to win at this whole diet and weight loss game? Do you wish that you could wave a magic wand and—poof!—Just like that your weight issues would be gone, leaving you with a body that feels healthy and that you would feel comfortable spending the rest of your life in? Are you like Lisa, in a sense, waiting for the weight to come off before you can live your full potential? Are you sick and tired of spending so much time on dieting and exercise just to find that you still hate your body?

What is it going to take for your struggle with your weight to end? How are you going to stop this struggle, this darn dieting and weight loss struggle that consumes your life? Is your weight always going to be the big elephant in the room? Or is it going to be the big wild elephant in the room that is talked about a lot, but you can't seem to make go away? Not that this is going to make you feel better, but you are not alone.

There are thousands of women going through exactly what you are going through, feeling stuck in what seems to be an ongoing dieting rut, full of heartache, shame, guilt, and disappointment—especially disappointment. You would think that with all the help available to you from the dieting industry you would not be in this situation and that there would be a lot less overweight and unhappy people in the world.

Could it be possible that there is something missing or something that we don't understand about this whole dieting and weight loss process that if we did understand, would change everything? I believe with all my heart that there is, and I would like to share this with you, along with the story of how my life led me to this understanding, which, by the way, did change everything for me.

The Pain Is Real

The story of how I came to be a weight loss and body image coach is kind of unique, but I hope that me sharing it with you will perhaps help you understand how, although our weight loss stories may be different, our search for love, acceptance, and freedom are all the same. I would love for it to inspire you to always listen to your heart.

Born into a Cult

I was born into a polygamist cult in Mexico, and I am one of my father's fifty-seven children from his eleven wives. I was brainwashed at the age of sixteen to marry my thirty-year-old brother-in-law, a polygamist man, as his third wife. I was taught to believe that the only way to enter heaven was through living a law called celestial marriage, also known as polygamy, and that a woman could never make it into heaven on her own; she needed a man to take her there. I believed both of these lies, along with many others lies, for what seemed like an eternity, but after listening to my heart and seeking truth for several years, I found the courage to flee this cult.

Standing up to my father and my then-husband and fleeing with my three children without any idea where I would end up was the scariest thing I have ever done. I was determined to follow my heart and to live the life that called me, a new and exciting life, a life full of hope, freedom, and self-expression, and the ability to make my own choices. The ropes and chains of restriction, control, and manipulation that I had experienced the first thirty years of my life in the cult were now gone. My life felt wonderful, and I loved being free. I was determined to not only survive but to thrive.

I started a successful million-dollar business while I went back to school, raised my family and dug deep into the studies of psychology and all things spiritual. Connecting with mind, body, and soul became important to me, and it didn't take long before I developed a passion for health and wellness. The gym was my second home, and everything about dieting, nutrition, and exercise became my obsession. I even got into natural bodybuilding and became a competitor. I had six different gym memberships at one time, not only for the variety of exercise equipment they each provided but for the many friends and people I got to know and to help along the way. Helping people became another passion of mine, and I decided that by owning a franchised gym, I could coach and encourage a lot more people. I also opened a small wellness studio.

Soon after, I began writing a memoir about my childhood and my experience with living in the polygamist cult in Mexico. I wanted to share with the world the bizarre lifestyle, the pain, and the suffering that I went through, but mostly I wanted to share how wonderful it is to break free from mental bondage. I taught my clients how to break free from their mental bondage and helped them to lose weight.

No matter whom I worked with and how much weight they needed to lose or not, I noticed their thinking patterns were similar. They all seemed to have much of the same feelings of guilt and shame about not meeting certain standards. Many of them were lost when it came to understanding food and weight loss, and each had a set of emotional troubles. I noticed that, although my dieting and workouts were based on bodybuilding, I could relate to a lot of what my clients experienced: restriction, control, obsessing over calories and macros, manipulating through exercise, good foods, bad foods, different diets, different eating methods, more of this or less of that and tons of guilt and shame when failing. I too would obsessively crave sweets and forbidden foods when dieting for a show and then binge on them when I allowed myself cheat meals.

Writing my memoir brought up a lot of yucky feelings from my past. Feelings of being controlled, held down, and manipulated again caused me to wake up in the middle of the night with nightmares—nightmares of me being stuck in a house (the house I lived in when I was in the cult) and desperately trying to get out. Although I knew that I was no longer in the cult and that I had freed myself from that lifestyle, I couldn't seem to shake the overwhelming feeling of lost freedom that followed me everywhere. I assumed that it was the writing that made me feel this way and that it would go away soon.

As I continued to diet, train hard, and work with clients, the feeling of lost freedom and imprisonment got stronger and stronger. By this time, I had finished writing my book, and why I continued to feel this way made no sense. I no longer felt happy and free as I had before. Foods, diets, exercise, and my clients' pain was all I could think about. I did not allow myself to focus on anything else, and I fell into a state of depression. Everything else in my life seemed to be put on hold. I felt like I was chasing something or running from something and that I couldn't stop until I got what I wanted. But I didn't know what that was. I spent months feeling this way deep inside. Over and over, people would come to me and tell me how I had helped change their life or what an inspiration I was to them. This only made me cry on the inside because they had no idea how lost I truly felt. I felt like I was back in the cult in Mexico and a prisoner again. But I wasn't, and my feelings made no sense to me.

Joining Another Cult

One night, I was startled awake by the same nightmare that I had repeatedly. Once again, I was stuck in the house in the cult in Mexico and couldn't get out. I sat up in bed, scared to death. When I opened my eyes, I thanked God that it was just the bad dream again. As I waited for the familiar feeling of panic to subside, I lay back in bed and reflected on this ever-occurring dream. Suddenly, an inpouring of understanding came to me. I immediately knew what my nightmares were all about. They were showing me that I had truly lost my freedom again, but this time, I seemed to have a choice in the matter.

I understood that I freed myself from the cult in Mexico but unknowingly chose to join another cult. This cult sort of promises heaven too, but instead of requiring plural marriage to enter the kingdom, it requires some sort of fitness or thinness. I call it the Thin Supremacy Cult. It's a cult that millions of people unknowingly belong to because they buy into and believe in its ideas, the same way I and my clients had—all of its ideas on what to eat, when to eat, how to eat, what is better, what body type is better, what is healthier, who is pretty, what it takes, who's accepted, who's not and on and on and on. All of my obsessing over dieting, weight, food exercise, and following all these ideas had imprisoned me. They had robbed me once again of my freedom.

Following My Own Guidance

I quickly realized that I had been going about this whole diet and exercise thing the wrong way, that I had been accepting and following a system without considering the brokenness of that system. I didn't realize that my body had all the answers I needed when I listened to it, that I didn't need—nor did I want—to permanently follow rules set forth for me by the Thin Supremacy Cult or the dieting industry. I started working with clients who felt trapped in an endless cycle of on and off dieting and weight gain. I used my process to help them heal their relationship with their body, with food, and with themselves. I taught them how to have both a body and the freedom they wanted by learning to follow their body's innate wisdom. Teaching this philosophy and coaching clients through this process is now one of my biggest passions.

If you are sick of being controlled by your weight and by endless unsuccessful diets, or if you can relate to the feelings of deprivation, food restriction, guilt, shame, disappointment, and unworthiness, I encourage you to read on.

Help Is on the Way

Perhaps you are wondering how the dieting industry and the Thin Supremacy Cult have anything to do with you and your weight story. Or maybe you can't imagine how this book can lead you to the point of keeping the weight off. I promise that as you read on you will see how, and the missing pieces to your weight puzzle will come together for you. The following chapters will take you on a journey that perhaps you didn't expect. As you find yourself making your way through these chapters, I recommend that you open your heart and that you allow yourself to dream, to hope, and to believe that you deserve what you are wanting because you do. There is a reason why you picked up this book. Although only you know what that reason is, perhaps one of the hidden reasons is so that you can free yourself from the hell you've been silently going through. All the desperate feelings to lose weight, the disappointment when the weight comes back, and the shame, guilt, and sadness you have been feeling no longer need to be a part of your experience.

The Miracle that Is You

You don't have to accept a life of being overweight and unhappy with your body. As you learn how to free yourself from what keeps you overweight, along with learning a new way to love your body, a miracle happens. This miracle is called you. You come through for yourself in ways that you never thought possible. It's sort of like what happens when you water a withering flower plant. It comes back to life, and it's able to experience itself as the beautiful flower it was intended to be. You are that flower, and by staying open as you journey through the pages of this book, you will understand just how wonderful of a flower you truly are.

You Deserve to Be Happy

A lot of people have a hard time believing that they deserve to be happy or to have a body that they feel honored to be in. Perhaps you do too. But this is so far from the truth. You can have it if you want it. It's a matter of understanding how, and it's a matter of listening and trusting yourself enough to make it happen. In the following chapters, I will show you how you can do that if you are willing to do your part and to integrate the ideas and concepts.

Taking a New Journey

I will take you on a journey where you will get to see how the dieting industry keeps you stuck. It looks at you as a victim and doesn't see how truly powerful you are and how truly capable you are of ending your struggle with weight. I will show you the power of your belief system and the power of your thoughts, and if you change your beliefs about your body, you will see your body change.

I will also show you how to stop letting body image control you and instead teach you the secrets to loving your body.

I will go into great depth on how to pay attention to and use your hunger scale successfully. I will also show you how to bring about necessary change and how to trust your way to a body you can finally love. You were not born to forever be unhappy in a body you don't love. It's important to remember this as you continue reading. Let's get started, shall we?

The Dieting Industry

As a whole, people in the United States (and a few other countries) are heavier than they have ever been. Obesity rates keep getting higher and higher, and self-loathing seems to be right behind. This causes me to question what in the world are we doing wrong? There has never been a time with easier access to the dieting industry's products, services, and procedures, yet people continue to get bigger and bigger.

Buying a Dream

It feels as though the dieting industry is all about selling you stuff that only offers short-term solutions. They sell you stuff that plays on your emotions of wanting to lose weight and to lose weight permanently. This industry knows how to tug at your center and how to tug at the part of you that longs to feel good about yourself. It doesn't matter how much weight you want to lose or how you try to feel by losing the weight. For instance, some people just want to make their loved ones get off their back about their weight. For others, it could be that they want to fit into an old pair of jeans, to feel healthier, or to feel sexier. For others, it could be as simple as wanting to be able to move around more easily. The reason doesn't matter.

The pitch that is used by the dieting industry is all the same. Do this, buy this, take this, and you'll get what you want—you'll get your weight-loss dream. Now, there is nothing wrong with dreaming about feeling better and doing something to help you attain that dream, but this is the dream that these companies and individuals thrive off of. Because you want the dream so badly, you succumb. They project onto you that they are your rescuer and you are the victim. You're the victim of body fat and food, and they will save you. And guess what? You believe them.

A Diet Can't Permanently Fix It

The real problem is when what you believe is the problem is not really the problem at all. Dieting for the rest of your life in order to maintain weight loss is not sustainable if you want to be happy and free to live. Some people may call this making a lifestyle change. Yes, you can make a lifestyle change and be effective, but what's even more effective is to make a belief system change that will make a lifestyle change not feel like hard work. Dieting will also never permanently solve your weight issues and give you the dream you have been chasing if you don't spend the necessary time to see how you got to where you are in the first place. What do you do once the diet is over? Usually, you go right back into thinking and believing the way you did before the diet started, and within a few months, the weight is back. Now you are back to facing another looming diet. It feels like an endless battle.

Switching out Your Lenses

What should you do once the weight comes off? How do you get your life back? How do you eat normally again and keep the weight off? These are some of the questions I want to explore with you in the upcoming pages of this book. I want to share with you how to view this whole dieting game through a different lens –a different lens than the one the dieting industry has you viewing it through, which may or may not be intentional.

I want to help you understand what's happening so you can now be aware and play the game your way. I want to show you how you can experience a diet differently. It's sort of like when I gave up believing in the God that the cult I was raised in taught me to believe in. I didn't stop believing in God altogether. I just realized that God was not what I believed and that I could experience God's love differently. It all happened by understanding and by shifting my perception.

Let's pretend that dieting is like going to church. Just because you no longer belong to that particular church doesn't mean that you can't still benefit by turning to and loving God outside of that church, right? This analogy will make more sense in the following chapters.

Constantly playing the dieting game is painful. Most of the time, it leaves you feeling like a failure when you can't lose the weight or when you do lose it and then gain it all back. It can also leave you chasing a dream forever as if you are chasing something outside of yourself and then living your life on hold for the day that dream finally comes true.

More Broken Dreams

For the majority of people, a permanent weight loss dream never does come true, like for my client Jeanne. She was in her late fifties when she came to me. She shared that she had been dieting since she was thirteen. She had spent almost her entire life feeling like a failure because she could never get there. She could never get the permanent weight loss dream that she had chased.

Then there are those like Chassidy. She was able to lose weight ten years ago and hasn't gained it back but only by staying on a super strict regimen. She came to me depressed and wanting help because she had hit rock bottom. She had spent the last ten years of her life in bondage by restriction and always in a state of fight or flight. This had her feeling stressed, depressed, and unhappy all the time. She didn't want to live this way anymore.

Now Amanda, unlike Chassidy, ate however she wanted to but never without terrible feelings of shame and guilt. She came to me weighing close to 300 pounds and was devastated. She binged on food all the time with a promise to herself that she would start a diet tomorrow or sometime in the future. That day never came as the weight piled on, and the feelings of unworthiness got stronger and stronger.

Three Types of Dieters

There are members of the dieting industry system who consistently diet to fix the weight gain (which goes up and down), and they are riddled with shame and guilt.

Then there are the ones who permanently restrict themselves. If they do eat off the plan, they find a way to purge the extra calories.

And then there are the ones who never diet but promise themselves they will as they too continue to eat with shame and guilt.

These are terrible ways to live.

Perhaps you can identify with one of the three types of dieters and are wondering how this game ever got started.

It started the first time you looked at your body and didn't like it. You decided that you didn't like what you saw or how you felt and that you were going to do something to fix it. You decided you were going to do some form of dieting. You had good intentions, but you didn't understand what was about to happen.

Feelings of Deprivation

Every diet has certain restrictions, from paleo to vegan to Atkins to low-fat to keto. You name it. You pick the one you're going to follow, and usually, you categorize foods into two categories.

Good food, bad food.

Healthy food, unhealthy food.

Allowed food, not allowed food.

Depending on what diet you follow is how you categorize these foods. No longer is all food just food with different levels of stimulating power. Certain foods are demonized. You tell yourself that these foods are bad. The problem with this way of thinking is that as soon as you tell yourself you can't have certain foods, you begin to crave them.

The other thing you are told from the dieting industry is that fewer calories eaten equals weight loss, which it does—sometimes—until your super wise body catches on to what you do and adapts to the lower calorie intake. (That's a whole other book.) Now, not only have you eliminated certain foods, but you also take in less than you did before. Both of these actions put you into a state of feeling restricted and deprived only because you know there is an abundance of food all around you. You feel entitled to it yet deprived of it due to restriction because you use the dieting industry's lens of victimhood (as in, "fat gain happened to me"); it makes you feel powerless.

If you lived in a third world country where you had to ration your food because it was scarce, you would not eat all the rations of food for a whole day in one single sitting. You wouldn't feel entitled to food knowing that it is scarce and hard to come by. You might feel hungry but not entitled. Feeling entitled yet restricted causes feelings of deprivation. Feeling deprived puts you in a stressful state. You live in a constant state of fear and under extreme amounts of pressure to restrict, and therefore, to deprive yourself when food is all around you. An essential human need is to eat, and in essence, you are fighting this need.

Abraham Maslow teaches the hierarchy of needs in which he places food as one of the primal needs of the human species. Essentially, you fight against your body's instinct to keep you alive. This is the reason why after a few days on a restricted diet you feel the cravings for food get stronger. It's not because you are weak-minded; it's because the body is letting you know it's going to die without food eventually. It has no idea that you are dieting. Your brain is wise and works perfectly when it flashes images of food in your head. There is not something wrong with you or something wrong with your willpower. This might be when you run to the dieting industry to sell you a product promising appetite suppression, which doesn't work if you're eating for emotional reasons anyway. Sooner or later, your appetite will win.

Appetite

Your appetite is one of the biggest blessings you have ever been given. Without it, you would not be here. When I hear dieting people curse their appetite, it makes me feel sad. They have not stopped to think of what a blessing it truly is. Have you ever felt horribly sick to your stomach and tried to eat something with no appetite at all? Can you imagine if you had to eat through that feeling for the rest of your life? Appetite means that your body is working perfectly. It helps you by making sure you get hungry so you eat and stay alive.

Deprivation and Overeating

Let's go back to the feeling of deprivation and the stress that this feeling puts you under. Everybody knows that being stressed raises our cortisol levels. It activates the "fight or flight" response that causes inflammation and wreaks havoc on our health. But not everybody knows that feeling stressed due to food restriction and deprivation is one of the big reasons why we overeat or binge on certain foods that we consider bad. I call this FR-PTSD (Food Restriction Post-Traumatic Stress Disorder.) You are unconsciously traumatized by your fight against food, a primal need that your body has to have in order for you to live. The stress alone from your fight against food is what makes you binge or overeat it.

The belief that the food is bad and that you can't or shouldn't eat it causes the FR-PTSD, which then causes you to frantically search for a way to soothe yourself or to move away from the pain. Food becomes the perfect soother. It's the aggressor (weight gain causer) and yet the soother all in one. This results in you constantly fighting yourself, in a sense, against your life. It's like living your whole life with someone holding a gun to your head. You are unconsciously the gun holder when you diet using the dieting industry's way of thinking, which is that you are a victim, that certain foods are demonized so you can't have them, and that your willpower is weak.

None of these are true. You are not a victim. Your willpower is not weak, and you always have a choice as to what you are going to eat. Human brains were wired to experience pleasure and to move away from pain as quickly as possible. You naturally want to experience pleasure, which food most certainly can and should help you experience, but you also naturally want to move away from pain, which food (through guilt and shame for eating it) most certainly can and does cause you to experience. This leaves you feeling permanently stressed and in conflict with yourself.

What about food cravings? A craving is the body's way of either needing to move away from the pain that deprivation causes (which eating the deprived food will do) or a way of trying to keep us alive by needing certain nutrients from that food, which, when in tune with your body, you will know. I will talk about this in another chapter. Remember, restriction is fighting your primal need for survival. If you didn't have access to very much food or if you chose not to believe that you are a victim, the feeling would not be that of deprivation. Now you might be asking, "Is it possible to ever diet without feeling deprived?" The answer is yes. It takes a few shifts in your perspective for this to be possible and these shifts are as follows.

You have to view the diet as a reset period and not a diet. View it as a way to allow your body to heal. View it as a period of allowing an abundance of health versus as a period of losing access to food. The focus should be on healing your body and not on depriving your body.

You have to really know and understand that you are absolutely not a victim of food or fat. I know this could be hard to hear, but without punishing yourself, you have to accept and own your choices. Weight gain is a natural result of eating outside of hunger. I will help you learn how to uncover your personal reasons for doing that, which are super valid, but you have to be willing to take ownership of your actions regardless. You have to do this without beating yourself up.

Next, you have to remember that food cravings don't happen because you are weak.

And last but not least, you have to understand that you do, always, have a choice about what you decide to eat.

In my experience, feeling deprived is one of the fastest ways to gain weight and one of the easiest ways to stay stuck in a dieting rut.

Thin Supremacy

Let's talk about another one of the deadly weapons the dieting industry uses to sell you their stuff. The ideology of this weapon is so powerful that it controls the minds of a ginormous amount of people. I call it Thin Supremacy. It's the idea that thinner is better. Where in the world did we ever get this idea? I don't believe the dieting industry knows. They only know that it helps them sell a lot of products, especially because they believe in this idea as much as we do. Why has our society allowed this ideology to have so much power over us? Who got to decide that thinner is better? All of God's creations are masterpieces. It's unbelievable how we have allowed ourselves to pick one body type to mimic. It would be like an eagle fighting its whole life to try to look like a flamingo or a duck thinking it needs to dedicate its life to looking like a swan. Ducks and flamingos and eagles and swans are all beautiful in their unique way.

Thin Supremacy as a Cult

Who put this ideology in the minds of people? This topic hits me straight in the heart because it's so close to home. It reminds me of the cult I was born and raised in, and I have named this ideology the Thin Supremacy Cult. In this cult, the key to heaven is fitness and thinness. In my upbringing, living celestial marriage held the key to heaven. I truly believed that I could not make it into heaven without a man, and I certainly would not be allowed to enter heaven unless my husband had several wives. I was even encouraged to help him find young women to marry. I was taught and brainwashed to live this law of celestial marriage when I was young without realizing that it was a bunch of bologna, the same way that in our culture we are taught and brainwashed to believe that thinner is better. People's belief in Thin Supremacy reminds me of this part of my past. We are not allowed to enter heaven unless we are thin or thinner.

I imagine it to be as though all the thin people (especially the girls) get to sit close to heaven in the front pew of the church. The slightly heavier people sit in the middle pews, not as close to heaven, dreaming of the day that they will get to sit in the front pews with the thinner people, and the super heavy people sit all the way in the back far from heaven. Nobody wants to sit in the front pews as much as they do, and nobody can understand how hard they have tried to be good enough to, but they can't get there because they can't lose the weight. They'll never be good enough, they believe. Ever. (Flamingos have it all, they think.) They just sit in the back and dream. A few curse the front-rowers, and others condemn the front-rowers, but mostly, they curse and condemn themselves.

This ideology unknowingly causes terrible suffering. A survey done by *Glamour* magazine showed that seventy-one percent of women feel fat while only forty-six percent are considered to be overweight, and an astounding ninety-seven percent of women are unhappy about a certain area of their body. If you could change this one area of your thinking and your belief system, you could live a much happier and more meaningful life.

You Are Beautiful

If you get nothing else from this book except the understanding and the knowing that you are beautiful no matter what shape you were born with, it will be worth it. My struggle to try and be someone else's idea of what I needed to be is what caused the most pain in my life. It caused me the most heartache and suffering. If you've had that same pain and suffering and this book can help you let it go, I will be honored. Whether you are a swan or a duck, an eagle or a flamingo, a creator that only creates perfection created you. The shape of your body is perfect. You are perfect. All you have to do is believe it.

Beliefs

Now that you understand more about the dieting industry and the idea of the Thin Supremacy Cult that we are all exposed to, let's talk about how you came to believe these ideas. The difference between you and the people who have been exposed to these ideas that don't care about their body or their weight is this: these people hear these ideas, but they manage to keep them outside of themselves. They don't integrate the ideas, but you on the other hand, along with a vast majority of others, heard these ideas and internalized them. You made them real by accepting the ideas. You bought into them wholeheartedly so to speak by saying "yes" to the idea enough times that it became a belief. A belief is just a thought that you keep thinking over and over again. You pick up hundreds of beliefs throughout your lifetime. Some serve you, and others do not, but for the sake of this chapter, I will talk about the ones that do not serve you or your weight goals.

Sometimes the beliefs you hold that do not serve you become unconscious. You may not even be aware of them. Thoughts like "Skinny people are born lucky" or "I'm safer when I have more weight on me" or "I'm not as good as that skinny girl, and I should deny myself food till I can be as good as her" may become unconscious because you internalize them and store them in your unconscious mind as a belief.

The unconscious mind is where all your beliefs are stored along with every memory and every experience you've ever had. It would be impossible to be consciously aware of all that is stored in the unconscious mind all at the same time. We store thoughts there that we can consciously bring up later when we need them. For example, what is your full name? Were you even thinking about your name before I asked you about it? Where did you have the memory of your name stored when you weren't thinking about it? It was stored in your unconscious mind, but you brought it to your conscious mind and into your awareness the second I asked you the question.

This access happens in a nanosecond. This is important to understand because decisions as small as whether to take an elevator versus the stairs or what to eat for breakfast (which can impact your life and your weight goals) will be made based on your unconscious beliefs.

If your stored belief is, for example, "It runs in my family to be overweight, so nothing I do will change that," then that belief might be what is secretly keeping you from taking the stairs or eating a different breakfast. It may not be that you're too tired or that you don't care about your health as you may have assumed. These beliefs are so hidden that you have no idea they are running the show or your life. You access a belief and make a decision instantaneously. You don't even realize that you're doing it. It's important to figure out what your unconscious beliefs are about food, weight, and your body because you are making choices every day according to these beliefs.

Beliefs lead to choices, choices leads you to actions, and actions lead to your results. Another example of an unconscious or hidden belief might be that "skinny people are just born lucky, and it's unfair." This belief might be used as an excuse to give up, to feel inferior, or as a way to tell yourself you're not good enough. You might even decide to be angry at the world, at God, or at your parents for this injustice. When the anger surfaces, you may choose to eat a whole bag of Doritos as a way of pushing the emotion away or as a way to distract yourself from feeling it. This is just another example of the sneaky ways in which unconscious beliefs unknowingly affect your life.

Choosing to Change Your Beliefs

Whenever you try to make changes in your life in any way and you are able to uncover the beliefs you hold that don't serve you, it becomes much easier to make those changes.

The interesting thing about beliefs is that it doesn't matter if they are true or not. As long as they are true to you, you will reap the benefits or suffer the consequences of those beliefs. Let me share another example of this with you. Suppose that you are standing outside with a friend talking when suddenly she points to the ground and yells, "There's a big snake! Stand back!" She believes that it's poisonous and that you're both in danger, so she runs to get something to kill it.

She comes back running frantically with the only weapon she was able to find: a rake. Her heart pounds, she breathes heavy, and her hands shake as she lifts the rake in the air. Fear is written all over her face, and her adrenaline is out of control as she yells, "Move, I'm going to kill it." She drives the rake down hard onto the snake, and it bounces up into the air and falls back on the ground with a light thud. Her fear turns to embarrassment. It wasn't a snake, she realizes; it was a stick that wasn't going to hurt anyone. She didn't know this at the time, and it didn't matter that it wasn't true. To her, it was true because she believed it. She had several physical reactions in her body, and she made several decisions at that moment based on what she believed, that a stick was a snake.

This is the same way that your beliefs affect you physically and affect the decisions you choose to make. The beliefs you hold about your body, food, dieting, and exercise cause you to make certain decisions. Decisions that may sabotage you in a way that you never would have thought of. Now, this is not something to be sad about because remember that beliefs are just repeated thoughts, and thoughts can be changed. But you do need to pay attention to and notice what thoughts you may be thinking that are sabotaging you and your weight. Helping people to figure out their story and their "not realized" beliefs is one of my favorite things to do. I love to see people's lives change as they change what they believe about their bodies.

What Are Your Beliefs?

A good way for you to figure out what unconscious beliefs may be sabotaging your weight goals is to pay attention to what you think when making certain decisions. Ask yourself, "What did I just think that made me choose this action?" Pay attention to your thoughts and feelings around eating and exercising and especially to your thoughts when seeing thin or heavy people. What you notice may astound you. You may have judgments or ideas that you would have never, ever believed you had. You may feel pity, jealousy, sadness, anger, or resentment. Just pay attention to the thoughts and feelings that come up. What do you think when you go to a restaurant, to a grocery store, or to a hot dog stand? What leads you to eat? What do you feel right before you eat? What do you think when you choose not to eat? What do you say to yourself when you exercise, and what do you say when you don't?

All of these kinds of thoughts have something revealing to tell you about your beliefs.

Thoughts Hold Energy

Another concept about beliefs (that are created by thoughts) that a lot of people don't know about is that they are made of energy. Have you ever walked into a room full of angry people and felt an overwhelming feeling of discomfort and tension, as if you could cut the air with a knife because it felt heavy and thick? Maybe you've walked into a room and immediately sensed the love and adoration of two people in love? This is because you sensed the energy and the vibration of the people's thoughts. Our bodies sense this same vibration, and our cells respond to it intuitively.

When you eat a slice of pizza or have a piece of cake believing that it is bad for you, then guess what—it is. The cells of your body sense and respond to this vibration. If you believe that having ice cream is bad for you and you have it anyway because you feel deprived of it, your body is going to respond to that ice cream in a negative way. On the other hand, if you have the ice cream believing that it is fine to eat it within hunger, then your body will receive and respond to it in a positive way. Medical conditions are a whole other topic and science that I can't possibly address in this book, but please do keep in mind the whole phenomenon of the placebo effect.

It's not the food, per se, that is bad like the dieting industry has you believing. Nor is it your body that is bad or broken for gaining weight. It's your body's response to you eating outside of hunger and the beliefs you hold about the food that keeps you from reaching your goals.

Body Image

Body image—what exactly is it? It's as the words indicate, an image of our body that we hold in our mind. What causes a real problem with body image is when the idea or image we hold in our mind doesn't match the body we currently have. This is what causes a lot of the suffering that most dieters go through. They typically get this image from what is portrayed in Hollywood and also from what they see, hear, and notice about their family, friends, and peers when they are young. It's how the ideology of Thin Supremacy that we talked about earlier got planted in them. The problem with this ideology is that it doesn't make room for all shapes and sizes.

Are You Using Body Image against Yourself?

You may think and believe that body image issues are not a problem for you because you are not trying to be perfect. Perhaps you've never wanted to be like a model. But what you may not realize is that you do use some sort of body image in your mind as a measuring tool against yourself. It could be the image of the body you used to have or the body image of a relative that's not necessarily thin. Even if you don't believe you could ever have a body like that, you still judge your own body according to these images in your mind.

My client Tonya hated that she wore a size 22W, but she informed me that she wasn't interested in looking like a skinny model. She just wanted to wear a size sixteen like her sister, Lorraine. When I talked to her about body image, she became defensive. She didn't believe she had a problem with body image at all because, as she informed me, she in no way wanted to be a model.

"Those girls look sick to me," she said, "and I never want to look like that." She assumed that because the image she held was of her sister's size sixteen and not that of a model, she didn't have a body image issue. As I helped her dig deeper, she came to realize that she did. She was constantly checking and measuring herself against her sister's size sixteen. She also uncovered that when she got around someone heavier, she compared herself and noticed that she felt better. She felt as though she was winning somehow, as if she was some sort of top dog because she was closer to her body image than they were. When she got around people who were thinner, she also compared—only this made her feel like she was farther away from the image, and she felt inferior. And when she found herself around people that looked like they weighed about the same as her, she felt relaxed and not threatened at all.

Remember what I talked about in the last chapter about this happening in a nanosecond? These judgments and comparisons happen instantly because of the unconscious beliefs you hold, your beliefs about thinness being better. This ideology is portrayed in commercials, advertisements, movies, doctors' offices, food packaging, social gatherings, and almost everywhere. We are bombarded with this ideology every single day. It's no wonder that we constantly try to measure up to it. It's the guiding post or measuring stick we use to judge whether we are succeeding or failing.

My idea here is not to teach you to fight against this ideology but to help bring you awareness of the impact you allow it to have in your life.

If by being aware of this ideology you notice that you have been spending your life trying to be a duck when you were born a swan, then you can make the changes needed to live a more fulfilling life; awareness is key. Don't allow yourself to ever feel unworthy again because you don't meet the image that society or someone else holds for you. This is a terrible measuring stick to use against yourself because it was not born from or chosen by you. You were born and raised in it, so to speak (like how I was born and raised in my father's cult without a choice). Now you can make the choice to find your truth about your body. You can learn to figure out where your weight should be according to you. You can figure it out according to what feels good to you and your body and not according to some standard set for you by someone else. I will teach you how to do this next, but for now, stop judging yourself when you are around others who seem to be closer to that image.

You also may have not realized that being a member of the Thin Supremacy Cult is partially to blame for your weight gain.

How so? When you look at your body and it doesn't measure up according to society's image (and now your own), you decide to do something about it. You decide to go on a diet. This is where the whole problem starts. This is where the dance or the game with the dieting industry began for you, the game that you never wanted to play permanently but that somehow you still play after all these years. You have fallen into the belief that you or your body are terrible victims of weight gain and that the dieting industry or something outside of you is going to rescue you.

Gaining the first amount of weight may have been caused by other reasons, which we will go over in the following chapter, but the judgment you placed on yourself by using the Thin Supremacy Cult's ideas and by choosing to go on a diet is why this whole weight issue continues to be a problem for you.

It goes like this:

Body image causes dislike.

Dislike causes a desire to fix it.

Fixing it requires dieting.

Dieting requires feelings of deprivation.

Deprivation causes PTSD about food.

PTSD causes more food consumption.

More food consumption causes weight gain.

Weight gain causes more judgment along with guilt, shame, and all that yucky stuff.

More judgment causes a desire to fix, and on and on it goes.

How in the heck do you rectify this? How do you stop this insanity? What are you supposed to do when you are overweight and want to lose it? Are you supposed to never diet again and stay overweight? Are you supposed to accept feeling unhealthy and unhappy forever? The answer, of course, is no. The solution is found through awareness and a shift in perception. Remember how I said that fleeing my father's cult and the belief in the God he taught me to fear did not mean that I had to let go of God altogether? I instead allowed myself to find the God that loved me and that encouraged me to listen to my heart. It's sort of like that with this. You can use a diet to undo the damage you may have caused to your body from all the years of playing the game wrong but not with the dieting industry's ideas that you are a victim and dieting is going to rescue you. You have to understand that if you allow yourself to feel deprived and you don't use your own measuring stick when you diet, you will forever be playing this game. How can you use your own measuring stick? I'll teach you how in the next chapter.

The Hunger Scale

Most anyone who struggles with weight and weight regain have, in some way or another, eaten without physical hunger or used food as a way to handle certain thoughts, feelings or emotions. This causes a lot of different health problems and can affect and create many types of hormonal imbalances that exacerbate existing weight issues. If we could all use our internal guidance system, our hunger rhythm to eat, we would be much healthier, both physically and mentally. Most of us know this, but we don't know how to do it.

Think of a newborn baby. Babies can show us how to follow a hunger rhythm perfectly. They never question whether the milk they are given is going to make their butts big or whether they should eat less because yesterday they overate. They don't look over at another baby that is eating and wonder if they should try that baby's milk instead because that baby looks thinner. They usually just eat when they are hungry and turn away from the breast or the bottle when they are full. (Granted, babies do need to suck due to their developmental sucking reflex, but it's not necessarily for the act of tasting milk. That's why pacifiers seem to work.)

It's the same way with animals. A cow never questions whether the grass it eats is fattening or whether it should be eating the neighbor's grass because it heard it was better for weight loss. Cows just eat intuitively. We stray from listening to our hunger rhythm for a myriad of reasons, and everybody's reason is uniquely their own.

My desire is for you to figure out what your reasons are. Once you figure out, understand, and deal with why you strayed and you undo the damage caused to your body from having strayed, you can go back to eating naturally and intuitively as you did when you were a baby—without fear, worries, or concern, once again deriving pleasure as intended and feeling at ease when eating when physically hungry.

When to Start and Stop Eating

The hunger scale that I use with my clients is from one through ten and is divided in half. One through five are the feelings of hunger with one being starving and five being no hunger at all, and then five through ten are the feelings of fullness with five being not full and ten being so full you can't move. Imagine it as a measuring stick that is up against your tummy with both ends hanging way past your midsection. The number five is placed in the middle of your tummy and is when you have no hunger at all but also no feeling of fullness. You're coasting at this number. The ideal place to keep your hunger is between three and a half and five, and the ideal feeling of fullness should not be higher than a six. This means to stop eating at five and a half because it takes a few minutes after you eat to reach the feeling of a six. Never, ever let your hunger go below three and a half, and never eat past five and a half. Even if the food is deemed good or healthy. That means to stop eating when you feel the hunger is gone and/or, depending on what you are eating, before your tummy's fullness reaches a six.

Food and the Hormone Called Leptin

We also get to keep in mind that no food is bad food or "fattening" food. Food is a form of fuel, which is measured by how much heat or heat units it puts off when burned with fire. These heat units are measured in calories. The number of calories a food has says nothing about its nutritional value. Some foods, like the ever-demonized food called sugar, have close to no nutritional value yet are high in calories, quick to digest calories that rapidly stimulate the release of certain hormones including leptin.

I don't want to go into a lot of details about leptin in this particular book, but what I would like to help you understand (so you can see why it's important to stay within the hunger numbers) is the effect it has on fat-burning and hunger. Leptin is a hormone that is stored in your fat cells and is released the minute you eat food. It signals to your brain whether you are hungry or not, and it also affects the fat-burning process that takes place in your fat cells. The more fat you have, the more leptin you have access to, which means it will take less food to stimulate the perfect amount of leptin. If you get too much leptin, the whole fat-burning process that your cells go through gets hijacked so to speak. It also gets hijacked if your leptin levels are too low. The right amount of leptin stimulation and the fat-burning process happens when your hunger is kept between a certain window or numbers on the hunger scale.

This is why two different people (one overweight and one not) can each eat the same-sized slice of pizza, but their weight is totally affected differently. The pizza was the same, but the people were not. Can you see how it's not the food that is bad or that makes you fat?

We have to look at all food as just food—some with more nutritional value than others, and some with more hormone stimulating power than others. But they all are okay to consume depending on the state of our body, our mind, and our goals.

Eating within a Fat-Burning Window

Back to leptin; sugar has high hormone-stimulating power, and if you have a lot of stored fat when you eat it, it won't take much for all your fat cells to release plenty of leptin. You need to eat a heck of a lot less of this food (without telling yourself it's bad or fattening) to stay within a fat-burning window. Otherwise you go past the window and guess what happens? Stored fuel. We have to mentally stop demonizing food and instead look at its stimulating ability and (depending on how we want to feel) its nutritional value. Sometimes the nutritional value may not be as important to us in the moment because our brain is seeking pleasure, and that's perfectly all right as long as we always stay within the window of hunger.

Checking in on Hunger

Notice if you tend to look for the feeling of fullness instead of the feeling of hunger being gone when you eat. You will end up overeating the highly palatable and sugary foods if you wait to feel a five and a half to stop eating, and of course, you will gain weight. It takes a smaller serving of these foods to make hunger go away (because of their stimulating power), but they won't necessarily fill your tummy to a five and a half. Tuning into your hunger is how you can allow yourself to eat anything that sounds good to you without gaining weight. When we make this shift mentally, we no longer feel like we are victims of food. We no longer cry, "You did this to me," but instead, we eat according to how we want to feel. We don't have to feel deprived of certain foods because we know we can have them if we want them when we are hungry—not emotionally hungry but physically hungry.

You don't have to put yourself in PTSD with food any longer. Somehow, just by letting go of the old way of viewing food and by taking responsibility for your choices (because you now allow yourself to have some), you'll notice after some practice that food no longer has the same power over you. You can notice how certain foods make you feel physically, and you can make food choices based on how you want to feel.

Looking at It as a Reset Instead of a Diet

I always have my clients practice eating to hunger for two full weeks before they go on any diet, except I don't have them call it or look at it as a diet. A diet has all the feelings of restriction that we have always thought of when we hear the word diet. I have them look at it as a reset period, as a way of resetting and healing their body from all the abuse it has been through. It's amazing how shifting your perspective from feeling restricted by a diet to feeling hopeful about healing your body can change everything. You no longer feel deprived, but instead, you feel like you are taking care of and loving your body. You can see that there is a light at the end of the tunnel.

Once the damage is undone and you apply the hunger scale form of eating to your life, you can live without ever dieting again. Each person has a different weight loss goal, so I don't suggest a cookie-cutter plan for everyone. What I like to suggest is that each person figure out exactly what his or her goal is and then pick a diet/reset plan that inspires them or that feels doable or comfortable. Some people may have a drastic amount of weight to lose, and some people may only need to lose ten or fifteen pounds to be at their ideal weight.

There are as many diet plans as there are fish in the sea, but if I was working with you, I would perhaps suggest one based on the amount of weight you want to lose, your body type, and the amount of time you are willing to put into healing your body.

Paying Attention to Your Emotions

During this reset time is when the biggest opportunity to heal your emotional relationship with food can happen. I encourage you to pay attention to the feelings that come up during this time. What are some of the beliefs, thoughts, and impulses that come up? Keeping a journal or notepad available is helpful. The best thing you can do that will give you the biggest result is to get curious and ask yourself why. Why am I feeling this way? What do I choose to believe that is keeping me stuck? Some people don't need to reset their body at all and can go right into learning the hunger scale. I have them do these exercises right along with learning how to listen to their body. Remember that the weight usually comes back after a diet because you eat outside of hunger. You believe that certain foods are bad, and you eat them anyway. You also believe that weight gain is your problem, but by now, you are beginning to understand that the weight is not the problem. It is a consequence of the real problem, which is eating outside of hunger. Whether you are eating outside of hunger because of your belief in the dieting industry's ideas or because you have not yet learned how to handle your emotions, you will continue to struggle with weight gain until you discover and resolve what your reasons for eating outside of hunger are.

Emotional Hunger versus Physical Hunger

"How can I tell the difference between emotional hunger and true hunger?" and "Why can't I stop eating at a six?" are two of the most common questions I get asked. The differences between emotional hunger and true physical hunger are these: physical hunger comes on slowly and has some type of physical sensation to it. Perhaps you'll notice grumbling or a slightly hollow feeling in your tummy. Maybe the back of your throat and mouth feel acidic or dry or different. Maybe you feel your energy level start to drop. Each person experiences hunger a little differently, but one thing to certainly be aware of is that it comes on slowly. Emotional hunger, on the other hand, comes on suddenly and all at once. You usually will have some sort of emotional feeling or a combination of feelings right before you make the decision to eat. Boredom, loneliness, sadness, excitement, anger, frustration, unworthiness, happiness, unhappiness, and thrill are just a few of the many, many different emotions that can be felt right before you choose to eat. At social gatherings, the feeling of wanting to fit in or of just going along with the crowd can also be an emotional reason for eating.

Our Brain and Food

Also, one of the main reasons for not being able to stop at a six can be because of something that was mentioned in an earlier chapter about how the brain works. Remember how you learned that one of the many, many functions of the brain is to move away from pain and experience pleasure? We derive a certain amount of pleasure from eating. This is most usually why people can't seem to stop at a six. The pleasurable experience of eating can be addicting. You may not be addicted to the food, per se, but to the pleasure you experience when eating the food.

There is nothing wrong with experiencing pleasure, but when you need it in order to escape or in order to fill a void for whatever is missing from your life, then that's when it becomes a problem. It's when you need instead of enjoy this pleasure that you get stuck.

The other reason why people can't seem to stop at a six is what we talked about a lot in chapter four: the feeling of deprivation. Feeling deprived will lead to overeating almost every single time you eat. It is pivotal that you change your mindset from feeling deprived or victimized to feeling in charge and like the decision-maker in your life. It is easier to make this shift in consciousness when you are no longer dieting/resetting or undoing the damage that you caused to your body.

The Three-Step Process

The way to keep the weight off is to:

- Overcome your reasons (all of them) for eating outside of hunger.
- Rectify the physical damage that this has caused to your body by doing what we now view as a reset period and not a diet
- And then reintroduce "eating to hunger"

Keep in mind that as the unwanted weight comes off through dieting/resetting, the body has to go through an adapting period. You have to give your body enough time to adjust to the new weight by slowly coming off the reset/diet.

You won't be perfect in the beginning, and it will take a few times of screwing up to finally get it right. But once you do, you will realize how much freedom you truly have when it comes to food. You will never allow yourself to be a victim again. You will stop letting food control you and instead leave your crappy relationship with food behind you. You must own your choices. After all, you do have a lot more say than you believed.

Tools for Tuning into Hunger

Here are a few tools you can use that will help you tune into your hunger and to use the hunger scale most efficiently.

Number One: As you find yourself wanting to eat, stop and search for where in your body the sensation for food is coming from. You will be able to tell if it's physical and inside your body or if it's coming from outside and you are bringing the feeling into your body. Notice if you feel it in your head. Notice if it's a feeling that makes you want to move away from it or if it's a feeling that is calling you to pay attention to it. You will be able to tell the difference between physical hunger versus emotional hunger when you pay attention to where you feel it.

Number Two: When you begin to eat, you naturally notice and focus on your mouth—how the food feels in your mouth, how delicious it tastes in your mouth, and all the bursting flavors you feel in your mouth. But when you try to decide if your hunger is gone, you need to pay attention to your stomach and midsection too. If you only ever focus on your mouth, you will only notice your stomach once you are too full and it's too late. While eating, keep going back and forth between focusing on your mouth and your midsection. I know this sounds ridiculous, but most people never scan their body for hunger or the lack of hunger when they are eating and especially not when they eat for emotional reasons because hunger is not what the emotional eater is addressing. It is the pleasure from the food in their mouth that they use to escape their emotions. How satiated, or full they are, is not important to them. Stuffing their feelings is.

Pay attention to your body during eating. It holds the answers that will help you eat within hunger like a pro or, better yet, like a newborn baby.

Number Three: Make a promise to yourself that every time you put anything in your mouth you will pause for a minute and bless the food. Also, bless the cells in your body that will be receiving this food. Imagine your cells jumping up and down and clapping their hands out of excitement for the nourishment they are about to receive from you. Sometimes if the choice of food you are about to eat is not what you know your body asks for, the simple act of pausing for a minute beforehand will help you be consciously aware of what you are about to do.

Number Four: Something that helps when you catch your mind flashing food at you after a certain unwanted emotion and you know you are not physically hungry is to ask yourself lots of questions. I call this exercise, "Questioning my way out," and it goes something like this. Is this going to help? Is making myself miserable by stuffing my stomach going to make me feel better in the long run? I know I might feel better at the moment, but how will I feel after, better or worse? Can I not handle this darn emotion any other way? Am I choosing not to handle this emotion any other way because eating is easier? Why would I choose this again? Am I going to keep pushing this feeling away with food? When is a good time to start loving myself? Tomorrow, which never comes and is not better than today?

Usually questioning yourself in this way will stop you from turning to food if you are truly ready to be free from emotional eating. Instead, you allow yourself to feel the feeling you are resisting or trying to stuff away with food. You allow it to come up by leaning and relaxing into it and allowing it to be felt is how you release it—not by burying it with food, which will keep you constantly overeating and overweight. As long as you are alive, you will have emotions. Embracing all of them is powerful. All emotions serve a purpose, but negative emotions carry a message. The message is either that the way you are looking at something needs to change, or it is a call for action. Knowing how to handle your emotions in a way that serves you instead of trying to eat them away with food will help you thrive.

When you heal your relationship with food, all other areas of your life will vastly improve.

Loving Your Body

As you see the dieting industry and weight loss game through this new lens, something magical starts to happen. You realize how much more control you have over your weight than you realized. You will no longer blame nor allow yourself to feel victimized. Nobody gets to tell you how you must look, what you must eat, or how you must act except for you, even though without realizing it you had given people this power over you. You did so by accepting and believing in the dieting industry's ideas and by unknowingly being a member of the Thin Supremacy Cult.

You now get to own the power to create that resides within you, which is your ability to choose. You get to choose what you eat, why you will eat, and how you will eat all based on how you want to feel. No remorse, regret, shame, or guilt anymore. It's simply choices that you choose to make and that you get to own. If you screw up, which you will because we all do and it takes practice, there's no need to feel like a failure or to blame your choice on someone or something outside of yourself. Give yourself grace by accepting that the choice you made didn't align with your goals and that you know you can do better. It's when you judge, condemn, and blame that you get pulled back into victimhood, but when you own and lovingly accept that you, and only you, are the one that made the choice and that you get to choose better next time, you can set yourself free.

Also, remember to check in with your emotional state. What were you thinking or feeling or saying to yourself just before you made whatever choice you made that you considered a screw-up? This will help you recognize if there's a pattern.

The Choice to Love Is Yours

Always make choices based on how you want your body to feel and not based on how the Thin Supremacy Cult says your body should look. Learning to do this will create a more loving relationship between you and your body.

Loving your body sounds cliché, but honestly, a loving relationship with your body is important if you're ever going to keep the weight off. Remember that thoughts are energy, and the body responds to this energy. If you are only ever condemning your body because of how it looks, you miss out on the benefit of appreciating all that your body does for you.

Appreciation Holds Magic

Appreciation is the quickest way to allow yourself to experience more things to appreciate about your body, such as weight loss, health, and vitality. Are their things you can appreciate about your body right now even if your weight is not where you want it to be? Things like your nails growing or your heart beating or your liver cleansing without you even having to pay attention to them? How about your body's ability to see or taste or smell or for your body's ability to take you places? What about the trillions of cells inside your body that know exactly what to do and when to do it in order to continue to give you life?

We have so much to thank our bodies for. When we realize what a miracle our body truly is and all that it allows us to experience, we are more likely to love and take care of it. When you look in the mirror and catch yourself hating or disliking something about your body, stop and think about what that body part does for you. If it's your thighs, then think of all the places those thighs have taken you. Picture what your life would be like if you didn't have them (thick or not thick), and then send them love. Thank them for always being there for you when you need them.

If it's your nose (that was one of mine), imagine your face without it. If not for your nose's ability to suck in air, you would have to permanently breathe through your mouth. Thank your nose and thank it for pulling air in for you without you even thinking about it. Do this every time you notice yourself disapproving of certain parts of your body. It may feel awkward at first to send love to those areas, but what you will be doing is changing the energy and therefore changing the way your body responds. Perhaps your nose won't change, but other areas of your body will benefit from the energy of love that you are sending it through loving your nose.

Is Storing Fat a Bad Thing after All?

Condemning your body for storing fat is sad. Your body works perfectly and does exactly what it's supposed to do with extra fuel. It saves or stores it for later use in case more fuel isn't available. Your body's fat-storing ability is a miracle. Try to imagine what your body would look like if it couldn't store any fat. Not good. Can you see now that fat-storing is not bad? What's bad is giving your body food that it's not asking you for, and the only way to know this is by really listening and paying attention, as discussed in Chapter 7. When you sit down to eat and your body lets you know through your hunger rhythm that it's satiated, listen to it. Your emotions may want you to keep eating, but your emotions have never been able to do the body's job, so don't continue to let them run the show.

Your emotions need you to pay attention to and nurture them in other ways and force-feeding your body when it's not signaling that it's hungry is not one of them. Love your body by choosing not to eat outside of hunger under any circumstance. Tell yourself that the food is not going anywhere, that you can always come back to it later, and that it will be here for you when your body is hungry again.

Bodies Thrive through Movement

Another super important way to love your body is to move. Our bodies were not made to sit at a desk or on a couch all day. Our bodies thrive with good blood flow. I recommend that all my clients find some form of activity that they enjoy and that helps get their blood flowing. Once again, don't let the dieting industry's ideas about exercise scare you or put you under pressure because you think you have to kill yourself at the gym. You just need to find activities that you enjoy. If it's dancing or skating or biking, it doesn't matter. Just move.

After trying many different activities, I found that lifting weights is my passion. I notice that I love feeling strong, both physically and mentally, when I lift. This is important to me.

I urge you to figure out what you are passionate about physically. If you don't know, try different things until you do. Sometimes you just have to try things a few times before you can figure it out, but one thing is for certain. Your mind needs to be in the game with you. If you feel victimized about this, like you have to do it or else you won't lose weight, you will be wasting your precious time. Movement is super important for your body, but you need to be able to feel how much your body thrives off of it.

Exercise Has Sparkling Healing Power

Something that I do right before every workout is to close my eyes and imagine my cells getting super excited about all the blood flow that is on the way, and then, every so often during my workout, I picture blood flowing to every single cell throughout my entire body. I imagine that the blood is loaded with magic sparkles that have healing power. These sparkles not only heal with their power, but they fill me up with light. This light feels so good. It washes away any struggle I might have with working out that day. It makes me say yes to exercise and yes to taking the actions to love my body. I understand that I can choose to say no and not exercise or that I could hate it and believe that I will always hate it, but I choose not to do either of those, and instead, I choose to keep myself in the game. Practice this simple mind exercise. It will help you stay mentally strong and focused.

When people ask me how I do what I do, I always laugh and respond with, "I've convinced myself that I love it," which is true. I literally chose to believe that I love it, and now, that belief is my reality. This is a belief that serves me. Remember that beliefs are just thoughts that you keep thinking. You can choose to believe that you hate to move or to exercise, or you can choose to believe that you love it. Either way, before long, your belief will be your reality. What belief will you choose?

Trust

This chapter on trust is not strictly for those of you who have already gone through the resetting stage and have learned how to deal with your emotions without abusing your body. A lot of what I talk about in this chapter is certainly geared toward that period of time after the process.

Most of us throw the word "trust" around without thinking much about it, but it's important to understand the feeling it evokes so we can teach ourselves to feel it toward our bodies. How does it feel to trust, and where in your body do you feel it? For me, trust kind of feels like a sensation of letting go, a surrendering. I can feel it across my shoulders and into my chest. It feels like liquid, and it's flowing.

What does trust feel like to you? Think of an object (such as a shirt and how you trust that it will cover you) or a person that you totally trust and access that feeling now. Close your eyes and tune into the feeling. Notice as many sensations about the feeling as you can. This feeling is the same feeling that you want to consciously create and feel toward your body.

Would you say that you completely trust your body right now, or do you try to micromanage it to the point to where it has lost its thriving state? Have you ignored your body by constantly abusing it to soothe your emotions, or has it had to create sickness and disease as a way to get your attention? Our bodies are wise and have an intelligence to them that is not comparable to any other machine. All they need from us is for us to choose to listen and to take inspired action for their good. They know how to get our attention, but sometimes we wait till we get sick to listen.

Our bodies have a natural genetic makeup and an optimal set point, so to speak, where they can thrive and function efficiently. We just need to trust our bodies and get the heck out of the way to allow this to happen. When we trust our body and we take inspired action, our body can lead us to the right food, doctor, book, or piece of information that will heal or keep our body well. Most of us have no idea what it means to trust our body, and that's understandable because we have spent most of our life trying to do what the dieting industry has told us to do. Or we have been trying to make our bodies match the Thin Supremacy Cults ideology. We haven't learned how to trust our body's inner wisdom and to accept the gift that it is outside of its image.

Your Body Has a Designer

Your body was designed and engineered by the best designer and engineer in the whole universe, and if you accept this truth, your life will change. How can you be sure about this? The sheer fact that you are alive and have life flowing through you is proof that you were created perfectly; otherwise, you would not be here. Do you believe that it is possible for infinite intelligence to screw up? It is quoted that we are made in God's image, and you being anything but perfect would imply that God is a screw-up as well. It's the social pressure of thin supremacy that has made us lose sight of our perfection. We didn't all come to earth to look the same. We came to be different, and being created differently IS what makes us each perfectly beautiful.

Do not make it your desire to be perfect according to thin supremacy's standards. Make it your desire to be exactly who you were created to be. You.

You Are Perfect

You can't trust your body if you can't accept that "God created perfection."

You can't accept your body if you compare your body.

You will continue to compare your body if you believe in the Thin Supremacy's ideology that thinner is better.

You will continue to believe that thinner is better when you can't trust your body.

You can't trust your body if you can't accept your body.

And on and on this vicious cycle goes.

What I'm repeating here is what I mentioned in the beginning part of this chapter—that your body was designed by the top-dog designer of the universe, and that it's beautiful just the way it is. You were born into this universe designed exactly the way you needed to be for this life experience. When you accept this truth, you will surrender to your body and trust it to do its job, and the best way for you to let it do its job is to listen to it.

Stop abusing it with your emotions and choose instead to consciously and masterfully love it.

Let Your Body Guide You

There will be times when trusting your body is painful, but you will be guided to make the choice to trust it anyway. For example, it may be hard to accept that when you're only eating inside of hunger your body decides to hold onto ten pounds more than you think it should. You have to trust that it knows what it's doing. As long as you know you are listening to it, you don't have to worry about micromanaging it. You don't have to go back to dieting and restricting food again, and you don't need to try and force it to drop those ten pounds by ignoring its hunger signals.

You can choose to trust your body's hunger signal just like you would trust its signal to pee. Do you ever think that you will not allow yourself to pee all day because you peed too much yesterday? That would be silly right? You pee without question when your body needs to pee, just like you should eat without question (within hunger of course) when your body needs to eat. When you're listening to your body, it's easier to trust it. I can't say this enough.

The Most Important Relationship of All

There's one more thing you should know about trusting your body. The relationship you have between you and your body is one of the most important relationships you'll ever have, and just as in any relationship, there needs to be certain qualities for that relationship to thrive. Trust—along with integrity, love, patience, and so on—is one of those qualities. One of the ways for you to get the most out of this life experience is to be able to be present and aware of what you are feeling. Having a good relationship between you and your body allows this to happen and allows it to happen on a greater level than you ever imagined.

You could spend your whole life being disconnected from your body and still live, but don't you want to feel what it feels like to be connected? Wouldn't it be wonderful for your body to communicate with you fully about the deliciousness of every experience? Learning to fully trust your body and all its inner wisdom can open up a whole new life for you, a life that is free to flow and to be expressed through you and your magnificent body. Without your body, you do not have life.

Trusting your body ultimately means to trust your life.

Trusting your life leads to trusting the Creator of life.

Trusting the Creator of life leads to surrender.

Surrendering leaves nothing for you to do but to be, to enjoy, and to love.

Who knew that your body could lead you to all of this? And all you had to do was trust it.

Time to Integrate

At the beginning of this book, I shared with you my story of how I came to this knowledge and understanding and how it changed everything for me. It changed my whole approach to weight loss, lifting, dieting, maintenance, exercise, health, and the way I viewed my body. The results I got and the results my clients got due to this new approach were beyond what I could have ever thought possible. The biggest gift to myself through it all was not only the transformation of my body, but it was in getting my freedom back.

I no longer was living as a victim or feeling punished by a system that seemed to be against me. It is my truest desire that it do the same for you. I promised you that I would share with you how to keep your weight off, and perhaps you were a little curious as to how that would happen. I'm sure by now you realize that what you thought was the problem was truly not the problem after all.

You learned that your way of thinking and of viewing the weight loss process needed to be different. You learned how important it is to change your beliefs because what you believe affects everything. You got to see how the dieting industry's ideas are only keeping you stuck and how important it is to stop giving the Thin Supremacy Cult so much power over you. You learned how to love and appreciate your body by listening to it and trusting it more. You learned all about the hunger scale and how to let it be your guide, and to recognize whether your hunger is emotional versus physical.

Now that you have learned all this comes the challenging part: implementing it. Yes, implementing it is where most people get stuck. There are a few common reasons why this happens. The first reason is that although you may have understood this information intellectually, you have not yet been able to internalize it. You are not able or willing to bring it into your experience through practice. You may have fears or perhaps doubts, or you may just be the type of person that has to take some time to process things first before you can decide to move forward with it.

Another reason is because of the fear of pain. It can be painful to have to deal with emotions that you have been using food to cover up or to run away from. It also may be painful to knowingly accept the responsibility of your choices rather than unknowingly blaming some outside circumstance or event for them. Either way, it can be painful, and a lot of people have to work hard to fully integrate these processes, mostly because they can't always see or understand their emotional reasoning and may need some help sorting it out. It takes focus to uncover our hidden truths and beliefs, but doing so will render the difference between being stuck and unstuck or between succeeding or failing.

Here are the four steps that, if I worked with you, I would encourage you to do.

Step One: For a full two weeks before starting a reset diet of your choice (I would recommend one to you based on your needs), I would have you practice eating within hunger. During this time, you will listen closely to your body, and also, this will be the period where you will do a lot of the emotional healing. You will practice, practice, and practice what it feels like to be hungry and to be satiated. You will practice eating the bad foods within hunger and without giving them any value at all. You will notice and pay attention to how your body responds to all the different food choices you make and take note of this. You will not condemn or judge. Just observe and take notice.

Step Two: Now you will do your reset diet, all the while using the mindset of healing the body. This phase has nothing to do with restriction and everything to do with healing the body. You are giving the body a second chance. During this time, you will take great pride in your body and in your ability and willingness to love it by helping it reset itself. If I were working with you, I would have you pay attention to your thoughts during this time. Make sure that they are never, ever about restriction or deprivation and only ever about choice, about your choice to heal. I would encourage you to incorporate whatever type of exercise or movement that you enjoy into this phase all with the same mindset of loving and healing your body.

Step Three: Take a few weeks to slowly ease off of the reset phase completely. Slowly add the foods you love back into your diet. You want to give your body time to adapt to the new weight. As you make your food choices (within hunger that is), remember to make those choices based on how you want your body to feel. Please do not fall into the trap of thinking that if the food is deemed healthy that it's ok to eat it outside of hunger. We want this type of mentality to be a thing of the past.

No hunger means no eating.

Step Four: There is no step four, but if you have a little more weight to lose, I recommend sometimes that you do more than one round of resetting. This is a gradual way of getting the weight off so your body can re-adapt to the new weight each time. When the time comes for you to permanently be done with resetting, you will be a master at eating within hunger, and your relationship with your body will be one of trust, love, and respect.

It is said that "when we change the way we look at things, the things we look at change." It is my belief that "if you change the way you look at your body, your body will change the way it looks."

Conclusion

When I went through my deepest struggles with following all the dieting industry's rules and believing in the Thin Supremacy Cult's lies, my soul felt like it was dying. This was such a familiar feeling because I experienced it often when I belonged to the polygamist cult in Mexico. Here I was ten years later, experiencing it again, and would have never found my way out if I hadn't acknowledged my suffering and if I hadn't found the courage to honor the feeling that something just wasn't right. The night of my final nightmare is a night that I'll never forget because it changed everything for me.

As the inpouring of understanding came to me, I could see clearly how I had given my precious freedom away the same way that I believe you have given yours away.

I would like to share one final story with you about a grown woman I worked with named Erica. When Erica was in her teens, she wanted badly to be accepted by her thin group of girlfriends. Like them, she too believed in the ideology of Thin Supremacy. She severely disliked her body because she was not thin like her friends were. This caused her a lot of emotional pain. She didn't realize back then what she was actually doing when she turned excessively to food. She didn't know that eating was her way of soothing her feelings of not being good enough. All of the excessive eating led to a lot of weight gain.

She decided to go on a diet (one of many), so she turned to the dieting industry. She wanted help fixing the damage and the weight gain she had caused to her body by continually eating outside of hunger. The dieting industry gave her many false ideas about how they could be her rescuer and helped her establish the belief that she was a victim. Years of dieting and feeling victimized left her feeling out of control. She felt like someone else had control over her, and this made her feel like a prisoner. She explained how she felt like a prisoner in her body and that after so many years of dieting she had no idea how to listen to her own body anymore. After working with me, she was able to see how she had fallen into a vicious cycle. She changed her perspective and was able to untangle the web of emotions that were only hurting her. She relearned how to eat within hunger and finally feels free in her body.

My wish for you is that you use the principles taught here in this book to change your perspective, to lose weight, and to keep it off for good. No more emotional eating. No more feelings of shame and guilt, and no more feelings of victimhood. No more deprivation. Only eating what your body asks for inside of hunger. No more emotional eating. Ah, I already said that one, but I guess it wanted me to say it again because it's super important.

Millions of people have unknowingly given their power and freedom away to the dieting industry, and millions more subscribe to the ideology of Thin Supremacy. I wrote this book to spread this awareness and to teach how to be free from these ideas. I want to help as many people as I can, including you, to take back what is rightfully yours. You were born with the freedom to think and believe, and you were born with the freedom to choose what to think and believe, including the thoughts and beliefs about your body. What thoughts and beliefs are you going to choose today that will give you the body you were born to thrive in?

Herein lies the secret to the success you have been searching for.

Thank You

Thank you for reading this book and for allowing me to share my ideas with you!

As a way to say thank you, I have a free video class for you that is a companion to this book. Go to https://VeraLaree.com, where you can sign up.

Also, if you need help with your weight struggle issues, you can sign up for a free consultation with me by filling out a request form at https://VeraLaree.com, or you can email me at Vera@VeraLaree.com.

Acknowledgments

Thank you to Angela Lauria as well as to David Hancock and the Morgan James Publishing team for helping me bring this book to print.

About the Author

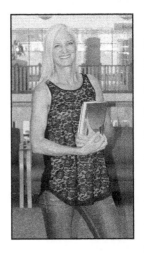

Vera Laree is a polygamist cult survivor and strongly believes in the importance of staying free from any system that mentally binds us. She is also a former natural body builder, a dieting industry rebel, and an ex-thin supremacist. She spent many years of her life devoted to the ideology of thin supremacy (which she likens to the cult she was raised in) and being at the mercy of the dieting industry.

She lives in Wisconsin, where she spends her time teaching her approach to weight management, weight loss, and diet-free living.

Her creative thinking ability has led to her dream career where she coaches individuals to also think outside the box when it comes to weight loss and body image issues. She holds certifications in therapeutic coaching, NLP, positive psychology, HNLP, and personal training.

Vera's ultimate goal is to reach the end of her life knowing that she inspired as many people as possible to dare to free themselves mentally from the reign of others, by thinking and choosing for themselves.

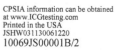

CPSIA information can be obtained
at www.ICGtesting.com
Printed in the USA
JSHW031130061220
10069JS00001B/2

9 781631 950049